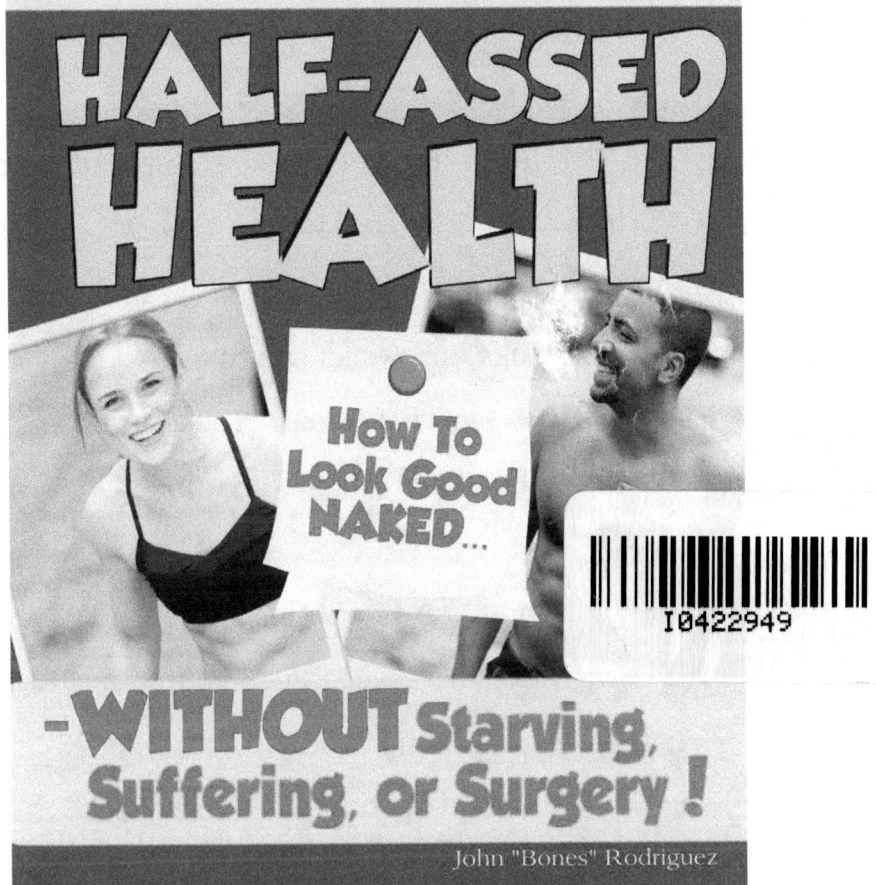

Forget About "Blasting Your Abs",
Shredding Your Quads", or "Ripping Your Pecs"-
YOU'RE NOT GOING TO DO IT ANYWAY!

HALF-ASSED HEALTH

How To Look Good NAKED...

-WITHOUT Starving, Suffering, or Surgery !

John "Bones" Rodriguez

HALF-ASSED HEALTH
How To Look Good Naked WITHOUT Starving,
Suffering, or Surgery!
By John "Bones" Rodriguez
2013 Edition Copyright 2013, Entreperformers, Inc.

Table of Contents

THANK YOU BONUSES

As a "thank you" bonus for buying this book, I'm giving you a few FREE GIFTS!

2 FREE Special Reports:

"The Obesity Conspiracy"
and
"The 4 Foods To Eat Before Bed"

and also several FREE WORKOUT VIDEOS!

"Better Than Burpees"
"The Perfect Breakfast To Look Sexy"
"The Hurricane Sandy Workout"
"Fat Dudes and Forearms"
"The ONE food you need to get Sexy"

Get them all at the Bonus Page:

http://www.HalfAssedHealth.com/Bonus

Thanks for buying this book, and please tell your friends that it's time to "Look Good Naked WITHOUT Starving, Suffering, or Surgery!"

INTRO: What the HELL are you doing?

There's no way you're sitting around counting calories and figuring out exactly how much you eat, and exactly how you're gonna burn off that cookie and all of that.

Don't you have a life?

Look, I get it- there are fat people everywhere, and it seems like it's really easy these days to get fat and ugly, and slow, and tired, and lazy, and as a result hate yourself, and get fatter and uglier, and lazier, and then hate yourself more, until you look in the mirror, and YOU don't even wanna have sex with you.

I get it.

I'm just asking what life can you have when you're freaking out about your weight? Freaking out isn't sexy either.

Most of us don't really care about the health risks anyway, we just wanna look good in our clothes so we can get naked, and look good naked too, and have sex.

I'm just calling it as I see it- I mean really- you're the one who bought the book titled "Half Assed Health", right?

Maybe you want to get healthy because you hear all of the great benefits of health, and have no interest in the "look sexy naked" part... Yeah.

In the fight between healthy and sexy, sexy wins, and fortunately, healthy and sexy pretty much go together these days... Pretty much.

If you're gonna go through this book and pick out all the stuff you don't agree with, then you'll probably stay ugly anyway, and no matter what I do to help you get sexy-looking, you'll still be ugly acting. So, let's just enjoy this time together, get the HALF-ASSED info, and get on with the lookin' sexy part!

Here's the usual pattern when someone gets a diet and exercise book:

Let's say someone wants to lose 10 pounds and burn some fat. Instead, they pick some crazy impossible goal, and get a "hardcore" book to lose 100 pounds in a month, and figure that if they only do 1/10 of the stuff in that book, they'll lose the 10 pounds, and then people will like then and then they'll be happy...

But I haven't really seen that work, have you?

So, now I'm only interested in what works- and what works for the life of freedom that I want to lead- nothing else.

I got sick of trying and training, and finding a new guru all the time, because all it did was leave me sore, tired, and frustrated.

Who the hell wants to be sore, tired, and frustrated all the time?

So guess what? I stopped going to the gym... BECAUSE IT HURT!!

Plus, who wants to go do THAT all the time? There are guys who look great, but don't have time or energy to hang out with chicks because they're at the gym all the time! What's THAT about?

Now, I'm not saying that you don't have to go to the gym, or that you don't have to put stress your muscles, I'm just asking what use is it to look good in front of the guys at the gym? And, of what use is it to be strong, but be sore all the time?

No use whatsoever! If you suddenly needed to swing from some vines and rescue a damsel in distress, you don't wanna be sore, right? You wanna be able to do it, and to look good doing it too... I mean- that's what I think about... doesn't everyone?

OK, so most of us just want to look better in clothes, so more people want to see us out of them. I don't know how old you are, but however old it is, it's just going to get harder to look good unless you start NOW.

I'm coming up on 40, and I want to make sure I start 40 at a good point y'know what I'm sayin'? So, I started a routine that wasn't such a big deal to begin with, and the point was to underachieve, and do it HALF-ASSED.

I had been underachieving in everything else, I figured, why not do it here too? My parents have been telling me that I do everything HALF-ASSED, but as far I could tell, everything has come out fine!

And if you know what I'm talking about, then you know that you've pretty much "gotten by" underachieving anyway, right? I guess if you have high goals. and underachieve, it's ok.

So here's the thing: you're going to learn to do the least work, for the most benefit, and do it all HALF-ASSED. Besides- you weren't going to follow those crazy routines anyway! Those routines make the fitness gurus more money because they know some "secret."

But they don't. Who the hell can do all these crazy routines all the time anyway? I often end up talking with someone who bought the latest "hardcore" workout DVD, or read about an "Insane" workout in Men's Health, but gave it up after a few days.

Those routines and diets aren't sustainable, they HURT, and they don't make our lives any better- they just empty our wallets!

Whatever I tell you to do, I'm doing it too. I like to be efficient and get things done as lazily as I can! Sometimes it's hard work being Half-Assed!

LEGAL- *Here to protect me from stupidity*

I hate that I even have to write this, but here goes: Before you undertake any new diet or exercise routine, consult with your doctor. I am not a doctor of medicine, or of sports medicine, or of voodoo medicine, and all advice is to be considered suggestions from an amateur who has attained results, and your results may vary. If you do something dumb, don't blame me.

Also, this is copy written, so don't steal it.

Like many of my other writings, I get to the point in this book, and do not bother to fill it with unnecessary facts just to fill up the book and make it seem like there's more value in it. I hope you appreciate the fact that I don't want to waste your time.

There's no need for me to take up pages and pages to write about what vegetables are made of, and where they're found if I really just want you to eat them.

Eat more vegetables! Done.

The fact is that the chapter "Counting" (which is only about 3 pages) is worth more than every other diet/exercise book you've bought before. Really- don't dismiss it. Everyone who has ever heard the idea has told me it is brilliant, and I concur... Now let's get to it!

AUTHOR- Who The Hell Is This Guy?

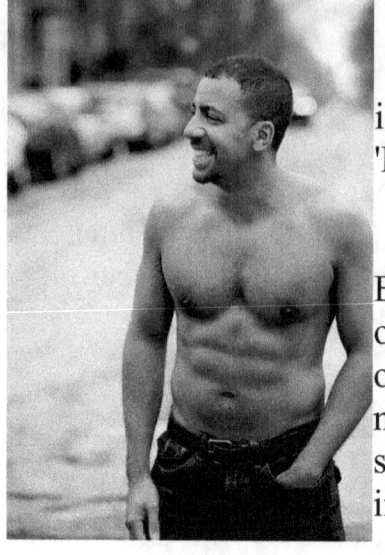

John "Bones" Rodriguez is the hardest working 'Entreperformer' in the world.

An Actor, Author and Entrepreneur, he performs all over New York City, and is often recognized from his national commercials, his short films, and improvisational comedy work

He is a graduate of The Bronx High School of Science, and earned his Bachelor of Arts in English from Skidmore College.

He has written several eBooks including "No More Waiters- How To Build Your Acting Business Without A Day Job", and "How To Make Money And Have Sex In The Same Room Everyday". In 2008, he released "Captain Kirk's Guide To Women- How To Romance Any Woman In The Galaxy" from Simon and Schuster.

As an Entrepreneur, he builds businesses online and consults others on how to do the same. The freedom of the "Solo-preneur" lifestyle is what he enjoys, and the website is dedicated to helping others achieve the same.

Having been skinny his entire life (hence the nick-name "Bones"), he began to learn about health and fitness, and worked to create the results he wanted. After reading a mountain of different books, and gleaning the critical parts, he then began teaching others to get similar results.

The skinny guys got bigger, and the big guys lost weight. They did the SAME things, and that was the big surprise... that shouldn't be a surprise.

Those lessons make up the bulk of this work.

http://www.HalfAssedHealth.com

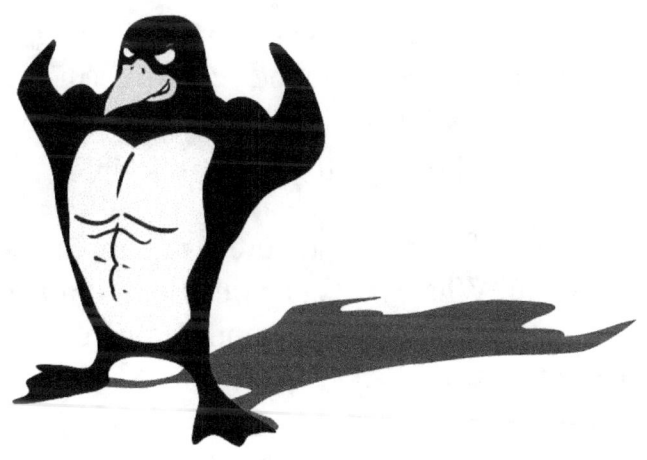

How To Look Like A Super-Hero

Here's your #1 rule for looking good naked:

People look better when their chests are in front of their stomachs.

Look at any drawings or pictures of fitness models, or of superheroes and heroines, and you'll see-the chest comes out, and they taper down to the middle. Women have a certain advantage here (well, some of them), but men have to work a little harder at this since we don't get boobs when we're teens.

And of you are a man and you DO have boobs, get rid of that stuff STAT- Boobs are for chicks!

I could make up some crazy ratio or a degree angle that would make this sound scientific (maybe some illustrations?), but you get the idea. Go to the mirror and look at yourself from the side and the front.

For some of us, it's a posture issue, for some of us it's a belly issue. Whatever it is, you'll look dramatically different when your chest is in front, and you're bigger on top than on bottom.

I could stretch this chapter out, with diagrams and stuff, but you get it, right? Good. Move on.

Why Goldilocks Is Sexier Than Snow White

Some people go to the gym everyday- some go once a week. Some sleep until someone kisses them.

The ones who go once a week aren't getting anywhere, and the ones who go everyday are definitely overdoing it.

Me? I have no use for going to the gym everyday. Gimme a break. Yuk. Disgusting.

However, I have realized that it'll do me good to go two, three, or four times a week, and there's a mountain of science says it's "just right".

(This is the Goldilocks reference. Got it?)

I TRY to go every other day, but that means I go a little less than that- sometimes I go twice, and on motivated weeks I've gone so many as 4 days. So TRY to go about 4 times, and usually hit three. Not too hot, not too cold, Just Right.

And NO- I don't keep a journal categorizing everything I'm eating, or what muscles I've done when, or whether I've done super-backflip-split routines with negatives.

It's a matter of "Did I go yesterday?" No? Well then I should go soon.... maybe today, maybe tomorrow... that's the extent of it.

Yes, there are days when I'm on vacation that I don't go that often, and there are days when I'm on vacation that I go very often. What I'm saying is that you can have a GOAL, and it's ok if you don't make it, as long as you ARE making progress.

So, let's say you go to the gym on Monday, then you can skip Tuesday, and decide on Wednesday if you wanna go. If you don't go Wednesday, you REALLY oughtta go on Thursday.

Again- that doesn't mean you sit around and do nothing all week, it just means you don't go to the GYM. I will likely take a walk, or maybe go play some sport, or I'll work extra hard during sex.

That's right, I said it.

That assumes you do some work while you're having sex. If not, I'm gonna suggest you get your lazy ass up and get to work. I'm speaking on behalf of your partner. And the other partners you're going to have in the future now that you're lookin' sexier everyday.

I recently moved a friend of mine (I'm 39, and still moving friends? I think it's time for new friends), and I made sure to work super-hard as we carried stuff up and down his 5-floor walk up. So, I considered that a workout day- I sweated a bunch, and my arms and legs hurt for two days. No need to go to the gym for a few days after that.

Speaking of stairs, I recommend taking the stairs instead of the elevator when you're only going three flights or so. I also recommend that you go up them 2 at a time. Just start the habit and stop bitching. A few years ago I made a New Year's resolution to go up stairs two at a time whenever I'm not carrying something too heavy, and I have stuck to it for years

It sure beats doing the stair-master for an hour! In NYC, the subways are underground (I'm talking about the trains, not the sandwiches), and there are times you can use the escalator. Instead, take I the stairs- even on 145th street where it's like 4 stories- just start this habit, and you'll see how easy it becomes!

You'll also get to see all the other people who should be taking the stairs just standing on a line spacing out on the escalator watch you as you zoom right past them and their flab.

There is an elevator at my gym (Seriously...*AT. MY. GYM!*) that I see people use, and that to me is WAY more than half-ass, that's just lazy! Taking the elevator two flights at the GYM is just ridiculous.

By the way, I've never seen any of the pretty people use that elevator.

Just keepin' it real, people.

Even BABIES Do This, What's Your Excuse?

I live in New York, where we kinda walk everywhere. This chapter may strike you with some fear, but babies walk at about 9 months, so you can too.

Look, if it's less than a mile, I'm walking. If it's nice out, and if it's less than 2 miles I'm walking.

Generally. Not as a rule, just generally speaking. Think about it this way- it's MUCH easier to look at good looking people in the street if you're walking. If you live in a place where everyone is fat and ugly, you should buy more copies of this book, and hand them out to people while you walk.

(That was my HALF-ASSED marketing pitch so you'll buy more copies, review and share this with friends.)

We all know that getting in the car is a waste of fuel, money, and not any good for your body or the environment, so walking is just a better choice. A simple, better choice to lookin' sexier that you can do.

I'm not talking about putting on your track suit and wearing a headband with a combination fanny pack just to get groceries; I'm talking about "hey, we need batteries, and the hardware store is about a 15 minute walk, so let's walk".

That's assuming you have someone to walk with. If not, you get out the music player, or audiobook, or teleseminar you downloaded, and listen on the walk.

You could also call up that friend you haven't spoken to in awhile; you've been meaning to tell them all about how great that "HALF-ASSED HEALTH" book you got is.

Or you just go with your own thoughts and figure out some problem, or let your mind go blank and meditate, enjoying the little details of life you usually miss. You may get some great ideas or inspiration.

Now I know that's crazy talk, and you might feel that it's a waste of your precious time to walk, but I'm telling you that if you're reading a book called "HALF-ASSED HEALTH" you aren't doing anything that important anyway, so you might as well walk.

You might also decide to take your bike out to accomplish some errands. Same deal, except you have an opportunity to look cool on your bike...

Unless you're on one of those folding bikes- those just don't look cool no matter what you do. But, better to be thin and sexy on an uncool bike, than fat and sloppy on an awesome motorcycle.

Most people are at a desk for several hours at a time, and that's not the way we were meant to live. Our bodies were made to be active, and if you sit in the car, sit at work, sit in the car again, and then sit in front of the TV or the computer all night, then you're gonna get old fast.

Physically and mentally.

Get out and walk- not the "race walk" thing, just walk more places in your life and see what's around- you'll probably like what you see. And if you don't like what you see- then change it!

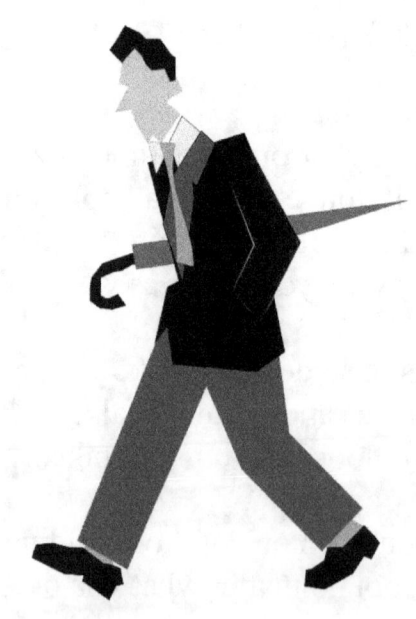

"I Want You For Your Triceps", Said No One Ever.

Since I don't go to the gym that often, and I sure as hell am not sticking to a schedule, or writing it in some little "workout journal", I am not going to try and figure out what body parts I worked on what days and all of that. Besides, when I tried that, I ended up always only working on the wrong thing, and being sore.

So you're not gonna do that either.

Who likes to be sore? What kind of "healthy lifestyle" is it to be sore all the time? Yuk.

So, we're gonna work out our entire bodies every time we go to the gym- a full body workout means you always get the right part in, and you never over-do any one part. Make sense? Yes it does.

There are people who are going to say that you "should" do parts separately, but in life, I never have to move something with just my triceps- just doesn't happen. So, instead, I do a full body workout, just like in real life.

The jug heads at the gym sometimes say "Hey Bones- if you don't focus on a body part, then you don't grow" they also say that you should be sore, and that's how you know it's working...

But check results.

Well, I look good naked, I'm not sore, and I have time and energy to have a fun life- doesn't that sound like a better way to live?

If you're going to get in a fight with a big muscle head guy, I'm gonna suggest you ask him what body part he worked on that day (or the day before), and then you can beat him up just by poking him in the right places- "Ow- My deltoid!".

Plus, since you never know for SURE when you're going to have to rescue that princess, or the orphans from the burning orphanage you want to be ready at all times. If you're sore because you "did biceps" that day, and you drop the puppies into the church fire, what was the point?

Also, if I'm gonna have some sex, I don't want to be all sore in an area I may need to use later on...

No- I don't work out my penis at the gym.

I do that at home.

But that's a different book entirely...

How'd we get here again?

You're a very sick individual.

The OTHER Organ That Should Get A Parade

Do you ever notice how awful alcoholics and drug addicts look? It's because they're taxing their liver. Your liver is very important, and we really can't live without it. That's why liver disease is so serious.

Your liver is vital- it does a bunch of stuff aside from fix your weekend drinking binges.

Your liver is the reason your body looks the way it does, since it cleans out impurities and "rust" from whatever you put in it, and then gives the body the materials it needs to grow.

Some people work out and have "Chest days" and "Arm days" so they can rest their muscles, but what they don't realize is that EVERY day is "Liver day".

And we should have a "Liver Day Parade"!

You get sore when you work out hard because your liver is cleaning out the acids from your muscles.

You need your liver, so be good to yours by taking days off from taxing it, and by drinking a lot of water to help it filter and process your food.

And don't eat ticker-tape.

Forget This, and You Might Snap

Like I said, I only like to be in the gym for a little while, so when it comes to stretching, I admittedly only do the minimum and I get it over quickly.

Some people stretch a whole lot, and can bend all sorts of ways, but I just want to look good naked so that's the priority. If I am feeling particularly tight, I'll do it longer.

Other people swear by yoga, and get all limber and bendy. I like to watch other people do that.

You know what I mean, right?

Yoga Pants.

Anyway, here are a few quick stretching movements that get your whole body limber and ready to go with minimal time:

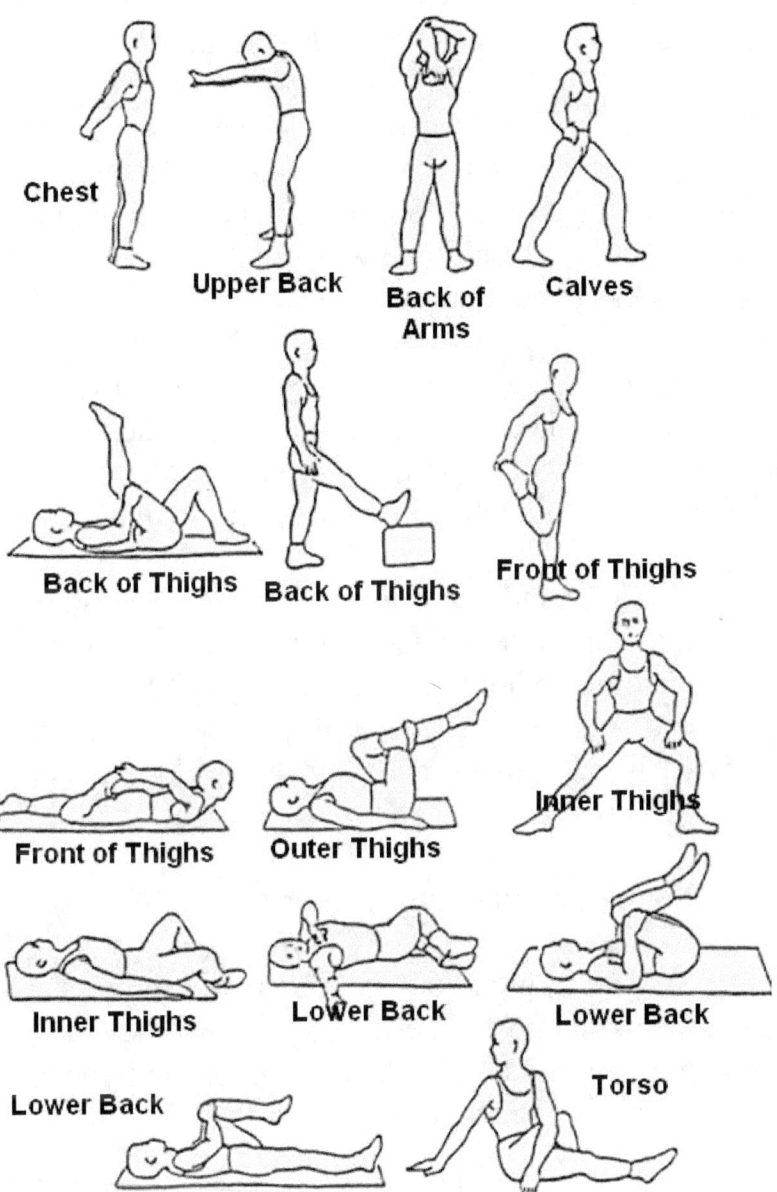

Chest

Upper Back

Back of
Arms

Calves

Back of Thighs

Back of Thighs

Front of Thighs

Front of Thighs

Outer Thighs

Inner Thighs

Inner Thighs

Lower Back

Lower Back

Lower Back

Torso

The Only Moves You Need For Maximum Effect

Every book I've read gives you dozens of choices for what exercises you should do, and the lets you "figure out what's right for you"... Well, if I'm gonna figure it out for myself then why did I need the 50 pages of exercises? I hate that.

So forget that- I'm all about efficiency. I want you to look good naked, to be able to do stuff, and do the least work to accomplish that task- I'm not lazy, I'm efficient. And I like the other things in life more.

I want in and out of the gym in about 30 minutes- including 10 minutes running time, because I got stuff to do like audition, shoot movies, do plays and comedy gigs, read books, write books, play video games, kiss my wife, watch movies, and save the world- and not necessarily in that order.

You've got other things to do too, right?

So, I've figured out what the main exercises are that get you the most benefit for the least time, and I'm passing them on. Just like the other books tell you, you will end up finding what works best for you, but on the next page are the 4 main large-muscle exercises, along with what body parts they affect:

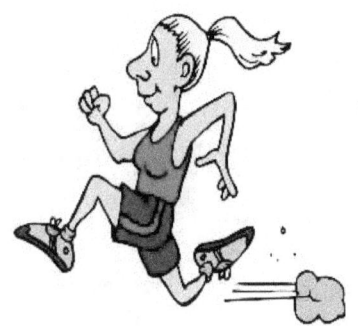

Sprinting
Legs, Lungs, Heart

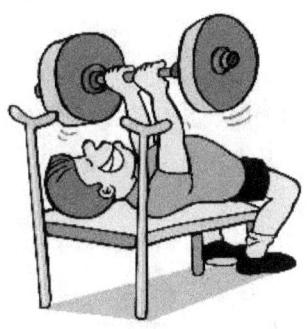

Bench Press
Chest and Arms
(and Ego)

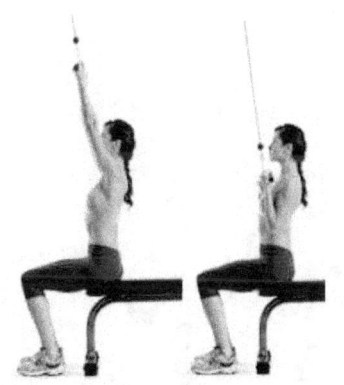

Lat Pulldown
Back and Arms

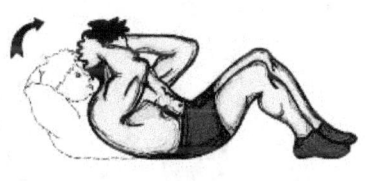

Crunches
Abs and Ego

"That's it? FOUR exercises?!"

Yes- because they are the ones that work the most muscles on your body. Now if you want to add to it (like I do), just for a little variation, then you can add these:

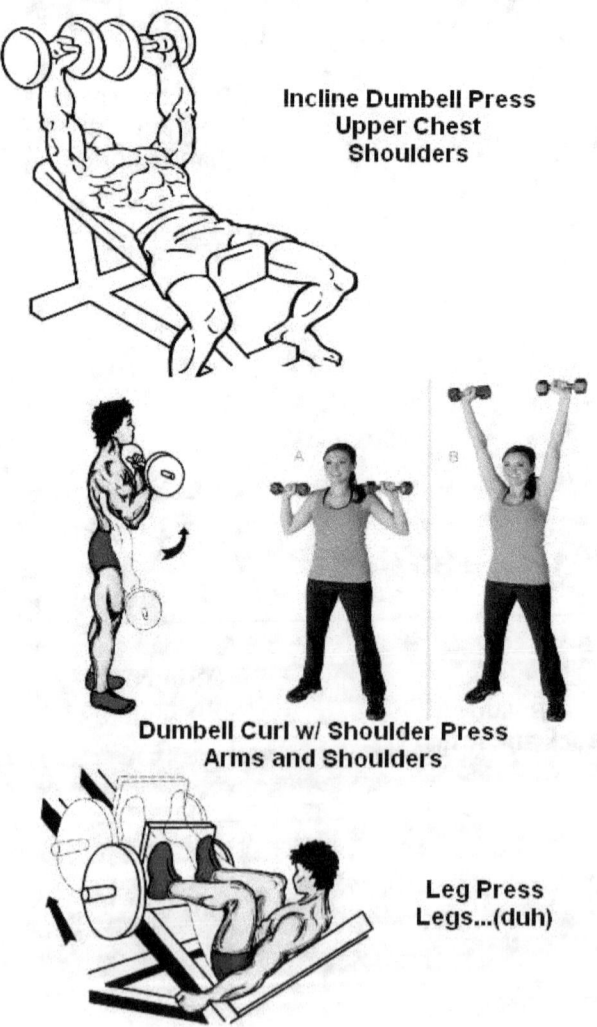

Incline Dumbell Press
Upper Chest
Shoulders

Dumbell Curl w/ Shoulder Press
Arms and Shoulders

Leg Press
Legs...(duh)

Add anymore, and you're cruising into AMBITION, and that is NOT HALF-ASSED. These eight will get your whole body done. Now, some people are going to say that if you just do that, you don't "confuse" your muscles...Whatever.

However, if you're one of these people who even know what the hell that means, then here's how to "confuse" your muscles: Sometimes do an exercise with a wide grip, sometimes with a shoulder grip, sometimes use your thumbs to grip the bar, sometimes don't, etc. Switch it around, but don't bother to keep track- that would be against the whole "confusion" idea!

I accept that some people <u>think</u> they need to do calf raises, or rear deltoid concentration presses (I just made that up, but it sounds real), and you can go ahead ambitious-boy; While you're concentrating on your minor muscles, I'll be out getting my drink on and lookin' sexy while dancing on the ceiling.

Honestly, I do 7 of those, leaving out the leg press, because I run, and don't see the point in doing more than that. I only put it there b/c everyone always talks about doing squats, but a lot of people get injured doing those. The running routine is good enough, bu if you insist, go ahead and do leg presses.

Doing forearms exercises is a waste of time. Doing Shoulder Shrugs is a waste of time. Do these 7 movements and get on with your sexy life.

What Are You Running From?

The thing with running is NOT to do a long, 30-minute boring run. People say they run for their heart, but you need to get your heart pumping FAST, not long.

One of the reasons people have heart attacks is that the heart isn't used to pumping hard, so what you're going to do is sprint and walk, sprint and walk. Pretty simple, you only set your treadmill for 8 minutes. The first 50 seconds, you walk (for example, at 3), and then you hit "interval", and you run (for example, at 8) for the next full minute.

Do that for about 8 minutes, and increase the speeds when it's too easy. I walk at 3, and run at 10 now. I'll probably stay there. If you run in the real world- like OUTSIDE (wow!), then use some measurement like a watch, or count your steps, or a set distance.

The next level of this is to sprint really hard, and then walk until you get your breath back, and then sprint really hard again for a few short bursts. Be tired.

It's not about distance, or time- it's about EXERTION.

You want your muscles to be trained with _explosive_ movements instead of the weak, low-intensity stuff. The difference between the body of a marathoner and a sprinter is all the proof you need:

Which body is best for health and performance?

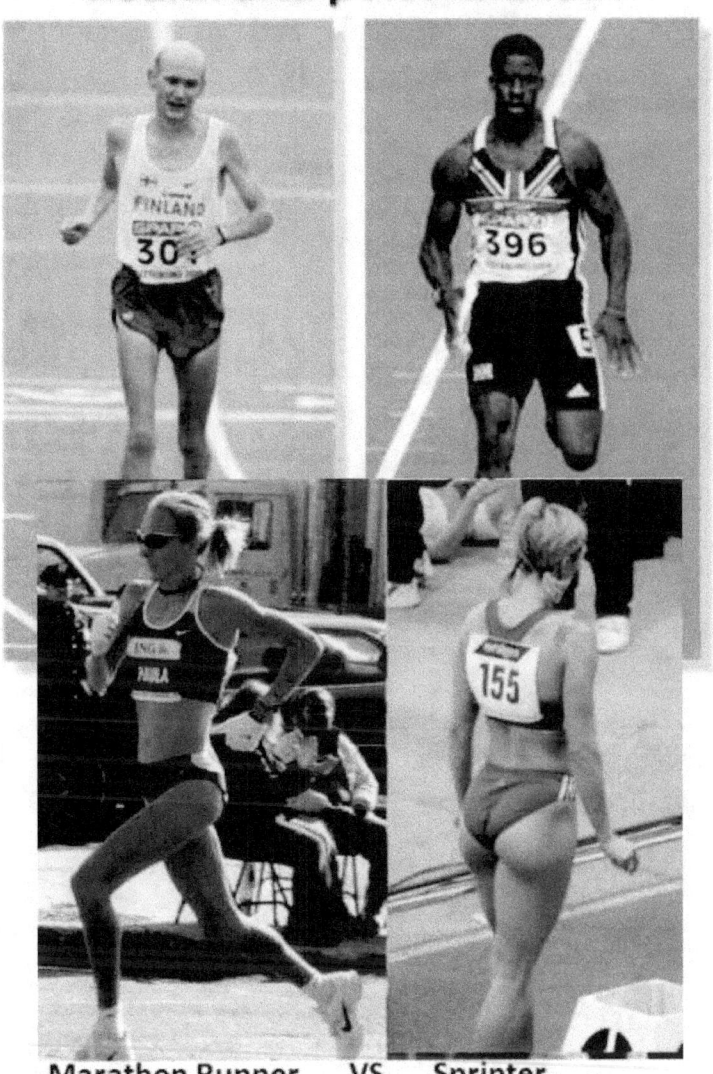

Marathon Runner   VS   Sprinter

The Most Powerful 7 Minutes Of The Week?

My wife and a bunch of her friends do Flying Trapeze (Yes, like in the circus), and are in amazing shape. When they're in season, my wife's fat loss is dramatic, and her back muscles give her a great v-shape.

So one day we decided to calculate just how much work she actually does when on the trapeze:

If each "flight" (as they call it) lasts for a maximum of ten seconds, and she flies an average of 15 times in a session, and she does that 3 times a week, then she's only exercising for a TOTAL of:

10 seconds x 15 times x 3 sessions per week= 450 SECONDS of working out, which is only 7.5 MINUTES A WEEK!

That's 7.5 MINUTES of exercise a WEEK, to have the incredibly fit body she has. Trapeze isn't a well-balanced movement, in that it is mostly in her arms and lats, but obviously her abs and arms get RIPPED.

By the way, she eats ice cream late after midnight, thinks cheese is a food group, and always has fries with her bar burgers!

...when they're in season.

When they aren't in season, she does some yoga, a little ballet, and she goes rock-climbing on occasion (I do none of those). The workout is very different.

Her body changes during this off-season, and isn't as muscular or ripped until she gets back to flying. She's still deliciously sexy-looking because her body is used to a certain amount of activity. Also sex with me.

The trapeze movements are **explosive movements, with short bursts of intense activity**. Look at the abs on this woman!

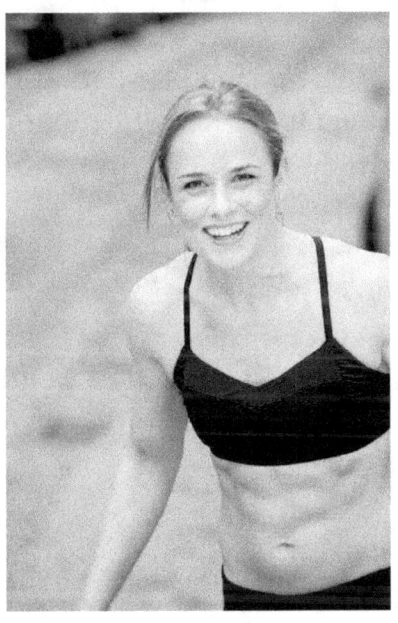

Think about <u>that</u> next time someone tells you they're going to train for the marathon to "get in shape". They are likely overdoing it, getting less results with more time, and straining their liver.

What Do a Bear and a Bunny Have In Common?

The HALF-ASSED HEALTH philosophy says that you always do a full body workout, but the question is what KIND will you do? There are only two:

"Bear and Bunny".

That's all you need to remember because there are only two things you're ever doing in the gym- lifting heavy so you can get "Strong Like Bear", or you're lifting light to be "Fast like Bunny".

I thought of "Bear", and thought it was cool, and "Bunny" just seemed to go with it better than "buffalo" or "barracuda". See? I'm even HALF-ASSED about how I name workouts.

Will you do a Bunny, or Bear?

Bunny means you'll lift lighter weights, a whole mess of times. Bear means you'll lift heavier weights, only a few times.

So, here's the rule of thumb: You always lift as many times as you can, but:

For BEAR, you lift weight until you can only do less than 12. If you can make it to 12, it's time to add weight. If you can only do 5, you have to take some off. More than 5, less than 12.

For BUNNY, you need to do at least 20. If you can make it to 30, it's too light. More than 20, less than 30. By the way- Bunny hurts more than Bear. This is another way for you to "confuse your muscles"

You also get the different "fibers" of your muscles, and blah, blah, blah- just do the two workouts. I just saved you a whole lot of time by not telling you all the science behind it. Just Do It.

Here's the thing- I said you don't need to keep track of what you do when, and you don't. Just in general, do mostly Bear, then throw in a Bunny once in a while. Like once a month or so. Yes- MONTH.

If you're working out at home, and don't have access to heavier weights, you'll do more Bunny. But you should really find a way do Bear once a week or so. Bear gets you the fat-burning results you want.

Note the "or so".. that means you don't freak out about it, you just remember to throw it in. Sometimes people ask me which they should do, and how often, and what percent of which, blah, blah, blah. Read this carefully:

IT DOESN'T MATTER.

Just mix it up between the two, and you'll be lookin' super sexy without obsessing about anything in your "workout plan".

The trick is to make sure you are always doing a full-body workout, and most of the details take care of themselves.

You need to engage your entire body so it releases all of the hormones and juices that get your body's metabolism up, and your muscles working and growing.

That way at any given moment, you'll be both strong like a Bear, and fast like a Bunny!

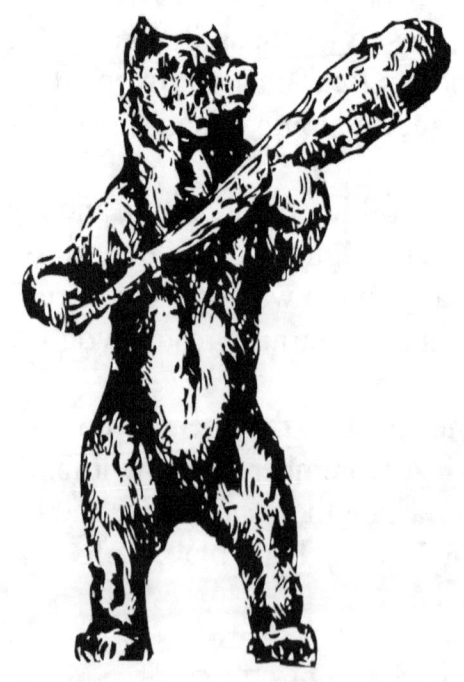

This is a bear with a club... he don't mess around.

The Most Valuable Chapter In Any Fitness Book You'll Ever Read.

Let me make something clear- this chapter is the highest value chapter in the entire book. This chapter is worth more than every diet and exercise book you have ever bought in the past, and is worth more than any money amount you can put on it.

You've heard of affirmations right? You know, those little positive sentences you say to yourself in the mirror or whatever to change your beliefs about yourself:

"I am beautiful, I am smart, and gosh darn it, people love me?"

Well- they're cool, but I invariably forget to do them, feel silly saying them, and my brain fights back anyway with things like "No you're not- you've got a big nose, you're a dummy, and if so many people like you, then why are you writing a book instead of hanging out at the playboy mansion?"

However, I'm all about trying stuff, so here's what I do. Instead of "counting reps" ('cuz that's just boring), I COUNT WITH AFFIRMATION SENTENCES! And you're gonna too.

When most people workout, they count from 1-10, and around 7 feel tired and barely make it because they know that they're close to the end- 10.

Instead, let's count with words that make us keep going:

I Love You What A Fantastic Day I Am Grateful

That's 10 words- get it? Look at it this way:

Nam
Myo
ho
Renge
Kyo

That's 5 for you Buddhist Chanters.

I
AM
BONES!
I
KICK
ASS
I
AM
GOD
AMEN!!

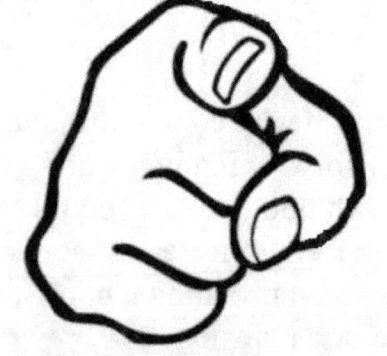

WHO IS THE AWESOMEST?
YOU ARE!

(For when I'm really pushing)

Can you come up with your own?

If I'm doing a bunny workout, I'll do it twice (maybe even thrice!) You're welcome to use whatever words you want; When I say "I Love You", I am actually talking to myself, the Universe, God, and YOU- because you are awesome and are reading my book!

You talk to whomever or whatever you want when you do your affirmations, but make sure they really make you feel energetic and proud to be you.

Make sure the more powerful ones are at the end; It's really hard to say "I am grateful" and not push those last few reps out.

Sometimes if it's really hard I'll say "Damn, I'm Sexy" at the end, or "F*ck You MUTHA F*CKA"!!! That makes it easier too... I'm from New York.

We talk like that.

All of us.

You talk to yourself however is comfortable for you, and throwing in a little funny can ease the pressure of trying to have that perfect body.

Some of the guys at the gym made fun of me at first, but lately I hear them saying motivating things while they're lifting.

They're still in there everyday, all day (I'm beginning to think they just want to sweat on each other), but they seem to like this suggestion a lot.

They don't quite say "I Love You", but you get the idea:

"Monster. Truck. Rally. Sunday! Sunday!

Sundaaaaaaay!"

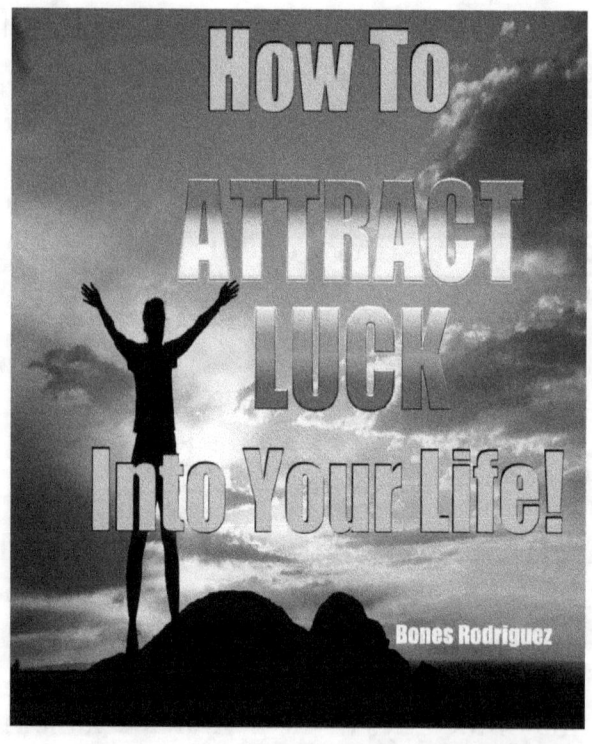

http://www.AttractLuck.com

Most People Do Too Damn Much Of This...

Most people eat too damn much.

Most people eat too damn much of the wrong damn stuff.

Most people eat too damn much of the wrong damn stuff too damn often.

Stop it.

Seriously- Eat only when you're hungry, or when you know you should. If you're one of those people who thinks they're hungry all the time, guess what- you cannot be trusted. You should then systematize it so you don't have to trust yourself.

If you are one of those people who eats too damn much- STOP IT.

You can figure out what you've eaten, and you know if you've worked it off or not. And if you don't, then eat LESS. There are a whole bunch of studies that say that animals who eat LESS than they're supposed to do better than those who eat more.

Something about metabolic efficiency or something.

That doesn't mean you starve yourself, it means you eat LESS than you want to. Eat some good protein after you workout like a whey protein shake, because protein makes you less hungry. When you eat meals, try to eat proteins with vegetables, or eat carbs with vegetables. Get it? Vegetables?

I read that when you mix your carbs and proteins that you stomach has to work extra hard to digest the two different substances, and you end up with poor digestion, which is counter-productive.

I didn't say to stay strict and drive yourself crazy about it, I said TRY to handle it better- Half Assed.

If you can get a burger with a salad instead of fries, do that. If not, then eat the damn fries- just not too damn much of the damn fries.

I'm going to suggest you look at food as the fuel for your body, instead of the fuel for your happiness. There are a lot of ads geared to teach you that eating equals happiness.

They are wrong, and just want your money.

Get the foods your body needs, and do NOT give it the stuff that makes it run badly, or that is actually poison. Yes, people sell POISON and call it food.

Which brings me to the chapter nobody likes, but we'll get through it quickly, and then move on, ok?

Sugar is Killing Us.

Sugar is a POISON to our bodies, just like alcohol or cigarettes are. And yeah, I eat candy, and yeah, I drink rum which is alcohol AND sugar at the same time, but not often. We have an epidemic of diabetes and it's because of how much sugar we eat.

Science has recently proven two things:

1. "Obesity doesn't cause diabetes: sugar does."

2. "It isn't simply overeating that can make you sick; it's overeating SUGAR. We have the proof we need: sugar is toxic."- NYT

Toxic means poisonous. Sugar is POISONOUS.

Read a blog post here: http://goo.gl/gLdoD

So stop eating all the sugar, and tell other people to stop SELLING all the sugar-laden poison and calling it a "part of a balanced breakfast." It's a lie.

A lot of cheap foods are filled with sugar and crappy carbohydrates, so if you eat like that be careful with it like you would alcohol.

Again, it's not to freak out and starve instead of eating a cheapo frozen pizza- it's to also eat something healthy with that pizza.

Snacks To Pack

I mentioned before that I like to snack on carrots, but I also have boxes of "PEELED SNACKS" around our apartment. They are organic fruit snacks with no added sugar or preservatives (you've seen them in a lot of stores), so I eat a ton of them.

I'm not really one of those "organic hunters", but they have these chewy dried fruit packs (mango is my favorite), so I just throw them in my bag and eat them while I'm out saving the world.

They also have these crunchy "apple clusters" that are almost like a crunchy cereal in little pouches. They are a great source of fiber, and have no gluten, dairy, cholesterol, or genetically modified thingys.

Since they have real fruit and fiber, Peeled Snacks don't give you the sugar crash, so they're great for kids, and I can finish a pouch in front of the TV without feeling guilty.

If I sound like I'm writing a commercial for Peeled Snacks, it's because I'm personal friends with the founders, and they hired my wife to showcase them on QVC... look how cute she is!

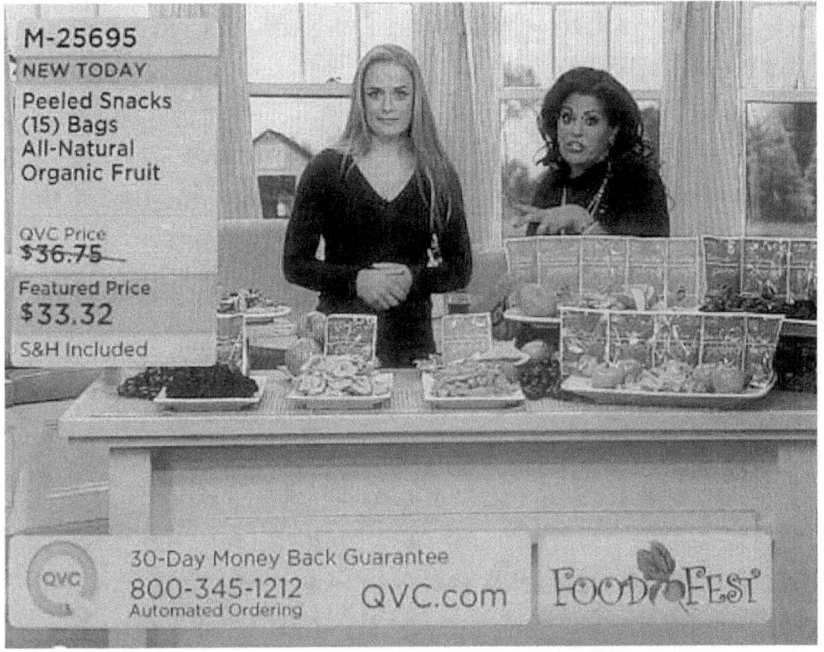

Peeled Snacks started in an apartment in Manhattan, and then went to airports, and now you can find them in some Starbucks', some Whole Foods, and all over the country. It's really a great success story.

I am super proud of them, the products are delicious and nutritious, so I SUPER-RECOMMEND Peeled Snacks!

To learn more and Order A Bag, go to:

http://www.PeeledSnacks.com

Making Your Choices Count Instead of Counting Your Choices

White bread is a bad choice, but I like sandwiches, so I TRY to have good breads instead. Like when I order from SUBWAY (the sandwich, not the train), I'll have the flatbread or the whole grain bread instead of the white bread.

It's not that it's a great, healthy choice, it's just BETTER than the white bread.

More often than not, we'll get the $4 "healthy" bread at the store, but if the "somewhat healthy" bread is two loaves for $4, we're probably getting that one. It's about making better choices, not freaking out over which is the "BEST" choice.

Like when my wife chose me... It was a BETTER choice than some of the guys, but probably I'm not the BEST choice... But that's for another book.

A lot of other gurus are always talking about making the best choice, but I want to tell you about just making the better choice.

Just don't bother eating white bread, because that's not made for your body to thrive, it's made for a corporation's investors bank accounts to thrive. It might as well be cardboard in a colorful bag.

Let's not reward them for their colorful marketing bags over rewarding people who sell actual food.

It's not that you should never eat pizza, but if you do get some pizza (and really, who can live without pizza?), then get vegetables on it. Broccoli, peppers, olives, onions (unless you're going to kiss someone), etc. Adding these make pizza taste better anyway, and you can feel like you're making a better choice.

If I go to McDonald's, then I get a grilled McChicken. It's not that I refuse to ever go, and it's not that I go all the time, but if I do go, I make a better choice, and you can too.

It's not that it's a great thing to eat, but it's BETTER than getting a triple-cheeseburger with bacon, which there is just no excuse for.

Except maybe a bachelor party weekend.

Whatever it is that you are eating, you can choose differently and simply make a better choice about it. It's not about being the food police, it's about making preferences based on what's good for your body instead of who's advertised better.

Like eating carrots over eating chips. Not all the time, but most of the time- and then HALF-ASS it.

A lot of parents are concerned with their kid's diets these days, and they should be. Kid's diets have been linked to several diseases both physical and mental. Why not take care of yourself as if you were your own child, and make better choices with your adult brain instead of the inner child's "gimme that now" brain?

And to talk about sugar again for a minute, I did a small experiment with myself and drastically reduced my sugar for about a month. I didn't have any chocolate, or ice cream, or any kind of "dessert" type of food.

I had no intention of quitting, just "pausing" to see what it would be like.

It was stupid! Also, I had crazy withdrawal symptoms, and it was a ridiculous thing to bother doing.

Except that when I came back to it, I couldn't eat as much, and I had NO DESIRE to stuff my face with sweets like I did.

Cake was TOO SWEET, and I could only have a little bit before I felt sick. So now, I have very little sugary sweets in my normal life, and when they do come up (birthday parties, etc), I really can't have a lot of it because I get full and grossed out.

Try it; reduce your intake and see how much better you can live without as much. I actually fully enjoy the experience, but on much less of it than before.

I will not be trying that with sex.

How To "Eat Right" Once and For All.

Why do you put your pants on in the morning?

Whatever reason that you have for putting on pants in the morning, you generally don't need to put them back on, or worry about where they are anymore, because you put them on already.

Your pants are already on.

Using the same strategy, I have a bunch of my "good food" in the morning at breakfast. Then I don't need to think about it anymore.

I already got the "good food" in.

For breakfast I have a fruit shake, with some juice, protein powder, and a "Scoop of Sexy" (I'll tell you about that in a minute).

I do that so I can check "Fruits" off in my mind, and I don't have to think about eating them anymore. It doesn't mean that I don't eat any more fruit in the day, it just means I don't HAVE to. I already got it in.

Fruits? Check!

I got that idea from Tony Robbins, who talks about having a "green drink" every day to get a whole bunch of other nutrients in one sitting.

That's where the "Scoop of Sexy" comes in.

Everyone knows they're supposed to eat a lot of vegetables, and shop organic, and chop your vegetables up, and eat a mountain of them every day, blah, blah.

But I'm Half-Assed. I want to do it once.

Like putting on my pants.

So, as Tony Robbins suggests, I started having a "Green Drink" which is how to get all of that good stuff all at once without the hassle.

A "Green Drink" usually comes in powder form, and it's a mix of all the great super-foods and vegetable concentrates your body wishes you had more of.

Plants like wheatgrass, spirulina, brocolli, spinach, and a bunch of other stuff you've never heard of that are fantastic for you, like eating "pure energy".

So, when the first version of this book came out, I was recommending a green drink from a popular store chain. Well, I met someone who loves this book, and is the CEO of a well-known vitamin company. He offered to create a special SUPER-DUPER Green Drink for me and my readers!

So, we got together, and looked at the ingredients of many of the other popular drinks, and grabbed their formulas. But we also took OUT all of the extra fillers, and added a few extra fruits to put it over the edge.

We also made sure to not add sugar that some have, and we came up with what I think is the best way to get all of your nutrition in one shot:

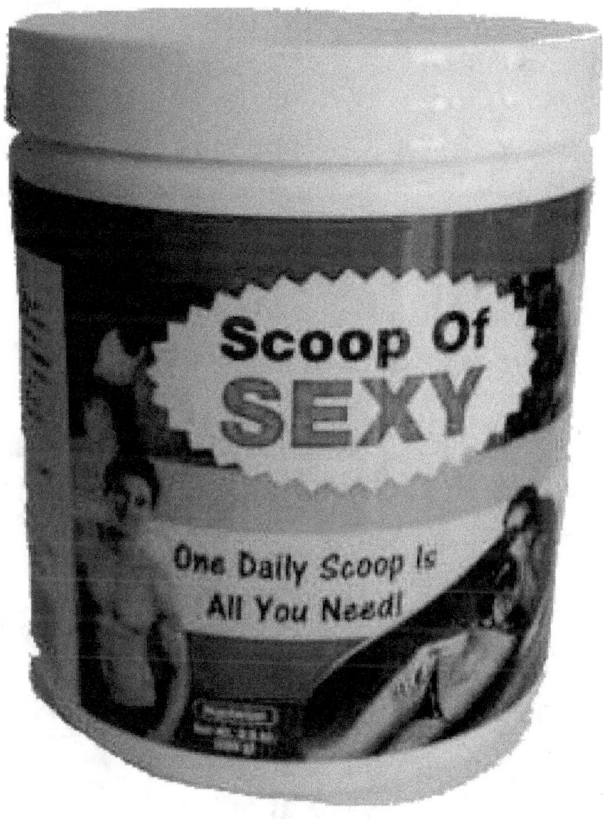

SCOOP OF SEXY!
(One Daily Scoop Is All You Need)

But why "Sexy"?

All of the other brands were copying each other with their "Green Blah Blah" and "Blah-Blah Greens", and I wanted my version to be SEXY, DAMMIT!

And "Green Sexy" was weird

And "Sexy Greens" was... weird too.

So, "Scoop of Sexy!"

Actually, it's more accurate than the other labels because the healthier you are, the more SEXY you are!

Plus, all of the greens are great for your circulation- which helps men... keep... up.... and helps women... feel... full.

The extra energy from the plants is sexy, as is the healthy benefits to your skin. All around, having this formula is really- A SCOOP OF SEXY!

You can learn more and order some SOS at:

http://www.ScoopOfSexy.com

or at
http://www.HalfAssedHealth.com/Nutrition

Next are some foods you should try to eat often:

Eat These Often!

1- **Spinach & Broccoli** You already know these are great.

2- **Yogurt** (I hate yogurt, and never eat it, just being honest) I eat a product called "good belly".

3- **Red Tomatoes**- You can just get a bag of those mini tomatoes and eat them in front of the TV. I also drink V-8 (low sodium) to cover this. Actually, when I go to brunch (we do brunch in New York), I usually ask for a ½ orange juice, ½ tomato juice mix. Sounds gross, but is delicious, and great for you- try it!

4- **Carrots**- Again, you can just get a bag of mini carrots, and eat them instead of chips. That doesn't mean you can't ever eat chips; it means that Carrots are a better choice. The truth is I eat a lot of pretzels, which are white flour and salt- but I have a bunch of carrots FIRST! They have a lot of sugar, but it's better than candy.

5- **Blueberries**- I toss these into my morning shake when I'm covering my "fruit" intake for the day. They have great antioxidants, and make you go to the bathroom, which is fun.

6- **Black Beans**- Ever wonder why Cubans are so smart? Well, black beans are good for your brain, and Cubans eat a lot of black beans! Eating black beans won't make you a Cuban, but you'll get all the benefits of being Cuban without having to be Communist! Yes, I am of Cuban descent... in case you didn't figure that out.

7- **Walnuts & Almonds**- The best of the nuts. Eat them unless you're allergic. Grab a handful before one of your walks, or whenever your hungry.

8- **Oats**- Doctors praise plain Oatmeal as a great breakfast food. The instant stuff has too much sugar in it, and that's why I rarely have any, but real oats have great fiber.

EAT A BANANA EVERY DAY - Because I said so.

But also, some people say bananas are almost the perfect food.

And they also make great comedy props.

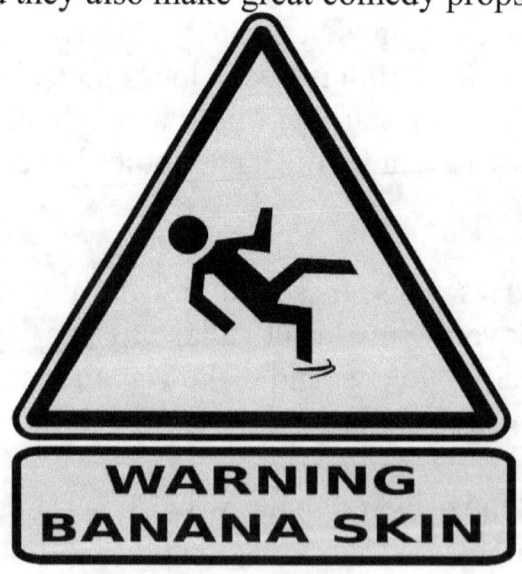

You're WHEY Better Off With This...

I have a lot of protein shakes, because I had my jaw broken in High School, and I suddenly had to have liquids only for 2 months. Then I realized how convenient it is to drink shakes instead of eating!

Whey Protein is great, but you really have to watch which one you use. So many of them have Growth Hormones from injected cows, and they also have the artificial sweetener Sucralose.

I really don't trust Sucralose; there are a bunch of people who are allergic to it, and it has some bad side effects that just don't seem worth it. Look it up.

So instead of buying the cheap stuff from the factories (that sometimes made me a little sick), I make shakes with the good stuff. Look for protein blends that are naturally sweetened with Stevia and that don't have the growth hormones.

If the label doesn't say "rBGH- and rBST-free", it's NOT!

My favorite is "BioTrust Low Carb", and I order it in special bulk from here:

http://www.Special.BioTrust.com

I also use it in a blog post video: http://goo.gl/ngVzg

EVAC- STAT!

I don't want to write this chapter, **butt** I have to. It's about evacuating stuff from your **butt**. What that means is that you should have a bowel movement twice a day.

Twice.

I know that you're probably not even having one, but ideally, you have three... Three? Yeah, I know.

Look, I don't want to be **anal** about it, **butt in the end**, your body should be making quick work of whatever you feed it, getting the waste out, and being ready for the next **load**.

If you haven't ever gone to the bathroom that much before, I promise, when you **load off all the kids at the pool**, you'll feel much, much lighter, have more energy, and feel strangely quick.

Just trust me that as you eat more healthily and exercise more often in efficient ways, your body will change to become more efficient and get rid of whatever is slowing it down.

This is not a load of **Crap**.

Winning The Mental Game

This is one of those chapters that people told me I should cut out because it makes me sound crazy. But if I didn't add this, I would be keeping a secret from you. Here's why I came up with this book:

In 2006, my wife and I went to California for 6 months, and while I was there, I decided I would fast. There's no scientific evidence that fasting is good for you, but that's what you do in California.

I fasted for 5 days, drinking basically just water.

(Note- I was supposed to have a special drink that I was supposed to make every day, with chili powder, and lemon or something, but as per my HALF-ASSED style of doing things, chose not to do that)

Anyway, here's the thing- it was way more of a mental ordeal than a physical hunger thing. On the first day I was hungry, irritable, and I had a splitting headache. My wonderful wife took care of me as I fiended for food like some crack junkie.

However, on the third day or so I got to the other side of the hunger, and I saw our entire world differently. That is to say that I saw how much of our lives are controlled by this never-ending desire to eat food, and how we can be unconscious slaves to it.

Being that I have a thing about authority, I hate feeling like I have no choices, and what I saw on that other side of my hunger was a previously-unknown slavery to our own desire for food.

I highly suggest you experience this feeling; it has never left me.

I could see how the food companies manipulate this natural desire in their advertising, and how our entire human existence is tied to our need for food and other basic necessities.

We really are animals.

It's kinda like after the first time you have sex, and you feel like a veil has been lifted from your world. When you realize that sex isn't nasty, dirty, nor is it necessarily all loving and soulful either. Whatever your pre-conceived ideas were, they often go away after having sex a few times.

Well, I felt like "Neo" and I could see the other side of the "hunger matrix". I'm going to suggest that you do the same some day.

On the topic of enlightening experiences, I have also gone out socializing with my eyes wrapped shut, and met many people while effectively blind. I only did it for one night, but it made a huge impression on me, and I've been meaning to do it for a longer period of time.

Whereas the blind experience was nowhere near the fasting one, I can recommend it as a first step so you might get curious to try the fasting one.

Again, there is no scientific evidence that says fasting is good for you.

Try doing without anything we normally take for granted for a while, and notice your life from the other side.

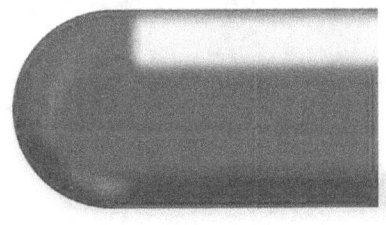

Red Pill or Blue Pill?

Do This, And Fix Most Of Your Body Problems.

Drink water. Seriously. Just fill up a Jug of water (64 oz.), and finish it during the day. Easy.

The BEST and most useful practice is to have a glass the first thing in the morning. You just spent 8 hours sleeping and not drinking water, so most people are dehydrated when they wake up. It's a BIG part of why you're groggy, but you don't hear about because coffee companies want you to buy coffee!

When I wake up, right before I shower, I drink 8 gulps of water. Making this one change will make an HUGE difference in your entire day.

I FRAKKIN PROMISE.

It's not that you shouldn't drink coffee- I really like coffee- I'm just saying that you should drink water first; it's a BETTER choice.

If you get up in the middle of the night to pee, drink a little water after that too. It's not about drinking gallons of water so that your bladder is about to burst all day, it's about staying hydrated.

Some days you'll do better with this than others, but when your pee is yellow, you need to drink more water. When it's clear, drink to keep it that way- that's a good enough measure.

CONCLUSION- Being Cute is Better Than Not.

There- that was HALF-ASSED Health. You can do that, right?

You can now go out and get sexy-looking without working too hard for it. Let's face it- it's just going to get harder, so you might as well get started now, and enjoy the process HALF-ASSED like.

We have a high divorce rate, and if you're a woman, you're probably better off staying in shape, 'cuz husbands and boyfriends really like cute in-shape women. If you stay looking good, then that will be one less thing for them to complain about.

And if you're a guy, and you keep in shape, you'll be way ahead of most. So you'll still be attractive to your wife's friends, who will remind her of that fact when she complains about you.

I'm just being real here, people.

And if you're single, then you're better off being cute rather than having to work so hard to overcome your looks with witty conversation. THAT is hard work!

I'm just saying: In today's world it's just easier to be a little cute, as long as you're not working too hard for it! Now go out there and HALF-ASS it up- you were going to anyway!

Can I Ask A Favor?

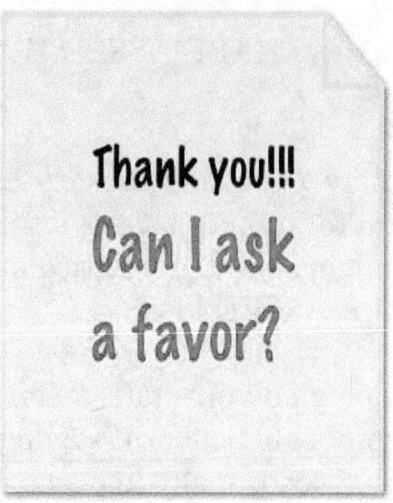

Thank you!!!
Can I ask
a favor?

As you probably know, many people look at the reviews on Amazon before they decide to get a book. If you enjoyed any parts of this book, would you please take a minute to leave a positive review for me?

You can do that here: **http://goo.gl/JHTP4**

60 seconds is all I'm asking for, and it would mean the world to me.

Thank you so much!

And don't forget your Bonuses:

http://www.HalfAssedHealth.com/Bonus

Please feel free to email me and let me know how you enjoyed this short report! I look forward to meeting you either in person, by phone, online- or by whatever the heck they come up with next!

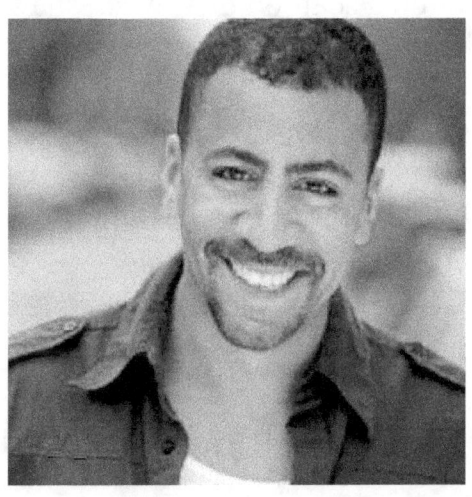

Let Your Light So Shine Before Men-

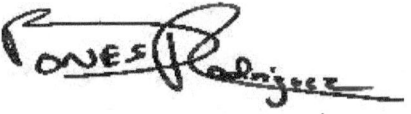

P.S.- Please, if you found ANY value in this report, please share it with your friends, family and social network.

P.P.S.- Don't forget to visit:

http://www.HalfAssedHealth.com

BONUS JOKES: YO' MAMA IS SO FAT..

When she steps on the Weight Scales it says...'to be continued'...

She once went on a seafood diet; when she saw food she ate it!

Folks exercise by jogging around her!

When she bends over, we enter Daylight Saving Time.

NASA plans to use her to shore up the hole in the Ozone layer

She was measured at 38-26-36 and that was just the left arm...

Small objects orbit her.

She makes Olympic sumo wrestlers look anorexic.

When I tell her to haul ass, she gotta make two trips.

When she farted she launched herself into orbit.

She lost a game at Hide&Seek only 'cuz I spotted her...behind Mount Everest.

She could be the eighth continent.

The only thing that's attracted to her is gravity.

Her graduation photo was an aerial

When she auditioned for a part in Raiders of the Lost Ark she got the part of the big Rolling Ball.

Her favorite food is seconds. Her belt size is Equator.

She eats Desert out of a Trash Can lid

She wears an 'X' jacket and Helicopters try to land on her

She needs a map to find her ass.

She fell into the Grand Canyon....and got stuck!

She wears an asteroid belt.

Her Passport photo says 'Picture is continued on next page'"

She's once, twice, three times a lady.

She was in the Daily Record last week on page 5, 6, and 7.

The circus uses her as a trampoline

Stunt agencies use her as an air mattress

When she opens the Fridge it says - 'I give up...'

She got a new gig at the Cinema...she works as the screen

She deep fries her toothpaste.

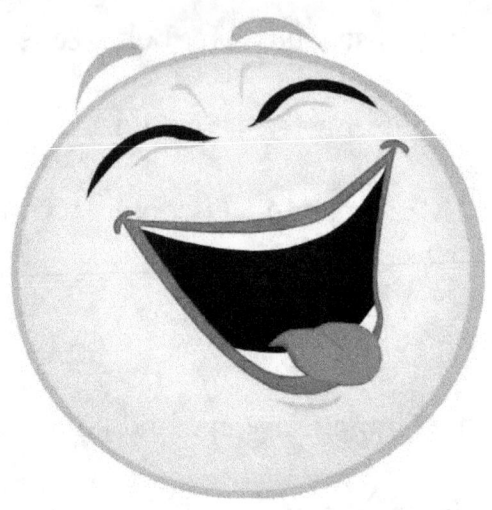

PUH-LEEZE remember to review this book:
You can do that here: **http://goo.gl/JHTP4**

60 seconds is all I'm asking for, and it would mean the world to me!

Thank you so much!

And don't forget your Bonuses:

http://www.HalfAssedHealth.com/Bonus

www.ingramcontent.com/pod-product-compliance
Lightning Source LLC
Chambersburg PA
CBHW060220290526
45789CB00003B/1338